I0423951

LOVING YOURSELF FIT

Achieve your dream body from within and love every step of the way

Meagan Mayada Hesham

Copyright 2016 Meagan Mayada Hesham

ISBN 1533190380

www.meaganhesham.com
meagan@rogers.com

CONTENTS

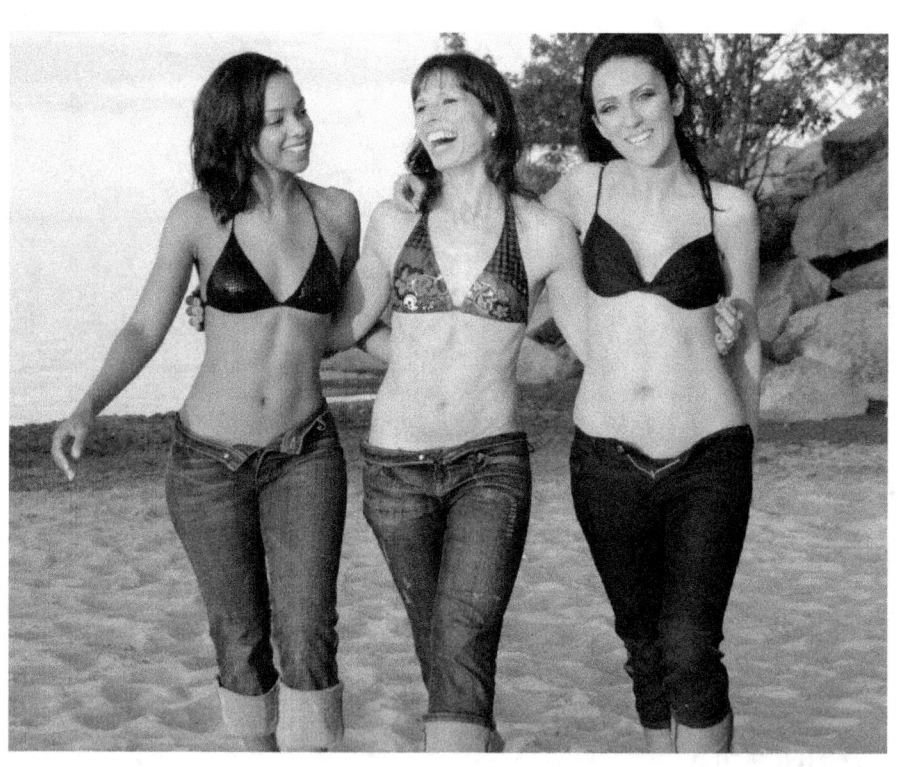

FORWARD

Congratulations on choosing "Loving Yourself Fit"! This is so much more than just a fat-loss book: the motivational, confidence-building, and goal-setting techniques you're about to learn will cross over to all aspects of your life. Once you've learned the skills you need to overcome any weight issues you may be dealing with, once you've learned to identify and manage the psychological reasons you cope the way you do – you will be able to overcome any obstacle holding you back in life, whether in money, career, relationships, and more!

Many people are aware of what they need to do to lose weight and be fit. Then why is it such an issue, such a daunting quest, for such a hefty percent of the population? The answer to that question – and the good news – the FIX – is the journey you've just embarked on.

People find it hard to follow through on resolutions made in earnest and the best-laid plans. It's probably happened to most of us at one time or another. Three things often stand between us and the success we hope to achieve: 1) mental roadblocks, 2) excuses, and 3) lack of smart and effective goal-setting. Most traditional fitness guides don't deal with these three stumbling blocks as often as I feel they need to. Sure they're full of solid diet and workout plans, even inspiring and appropriate quotes and bits of popular wisdom to try to point you towards your goal. There are hundreds – probably thousands – of books out there that can educate you on those things (chances are you've read a bunch of them already, and still aren't at your goal). So in this book, you won't find many specific eating or exercise plans…

I want to spend most of our time focusing on the really IMPORTANT stuff. Those three things I mentioned that are the real root of what's keeping you from your weight and well-being success. Ready to tackle that key part of your quest? Let's go!

WHO AM I AND WHY LISTEN TO ME?

I have been seriously involved in the fitness world in various capacities for over nineteen years. Over this time I've worked as a personal trainer, group fitness instructor, professional dancer, nutrition counsellor, and fitness studio owner. My love affair with dance started back in my childhood when I took classes at a community center, later performing with a troupe at summer festivals and community events. I've continued dancing, focusing at different times on tap, Highland dance, hip-hop, Latin, Brazilian, and bellydance. In high school my mom surprised me with a membership for us both at the local YMCA. I quickly became totally addicted to spending time there – working out with the weights, running, playing soccer, swimming, taking aerobics and aquafit classes. That's where I took my first fitness leadership course and then started instructing there myself. In high school I remember always wanting to lose those last pesky 5 – 10 pounds; I didn't want to be the 'big' girl. I exercised at home to a Jane Fonda workout video almost every day. I never lost a pound, though, because I would never give up all the junk food I loved so much. When I was about sixteen, I started taking bellydance classes. I started for something fun and different to do, never in my wildest dreams thinking beyond that. Was I ever wrong! I vastly underestimated the power of this empowering women's dance. I became obsessed with improving my dancing, delving deeper into the bigger bellydance scene in Toronto, and starting to perform with an amateur dance troupe. My hours of study and practice soon paid off, and my teacher began inviting me to do professional group and solo shows. And soon I was out there, performing all over town… with a big bare belly! I can't tell you how great bellydance and surrounding yourself with a culture like the Arabic culture is for your body image. All of a sudden you're being praised for your feminine curves! And just like that, it seems, my career as a professional full-time bellydancer was under way. But I couldn't ignore my passion for fitness and throughout the years I took on various part-time jobs in gyms and recreation facilities.

In 2003, I opened my own dance and fitness studio, Fierce Fitness, merging my two loves - fitness and dance. Teaching over twenty bellydance classes a week really taught me a lot about women's body image, weight issues, and what could be holding them back from so much in life, including achieving the body of their dreams. A lot of what I heard was very depressing to me – and this is exactly what eventually spurred me on to write this book. I believe anyone, no matter what obstacles they face, can get the body of their dreams (whatever that means to them personally). I'm not going to make any crazy promises or tell you it will be easy, because quite frankly, it won't. Anything truly worthwhile takes a lot of hard work. Depending on your goals this may be one of the biggest things you achieve in your life! So no, it won't be easy, but it will be worth it!

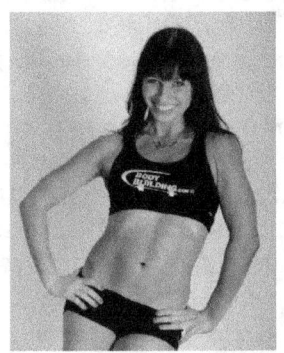 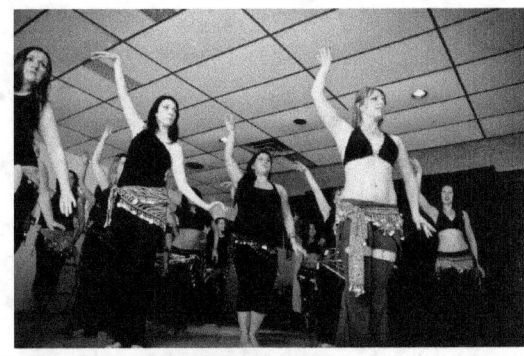

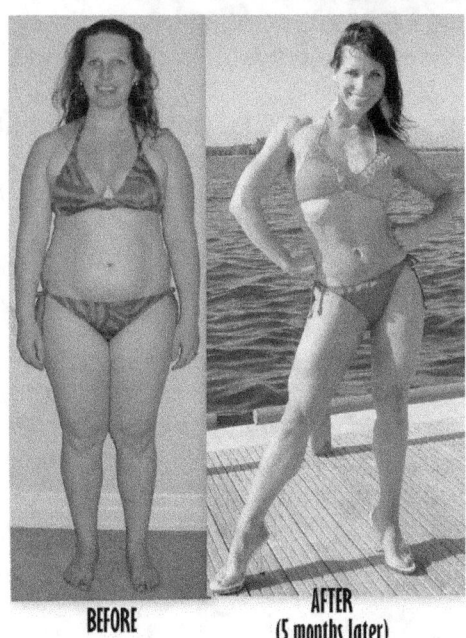

BEFORE

AFTER
(5 months later)

WHAT DO YOU REALLY WANT?

North America has a strange obsession with one ideal body type for women. A few years ago the body everyone seemed to lust after was the stick-thin runway-model look. Now everyone's loving the "curvy" (but not too curvy) look that's often achieved through plastic surgery - butt implants, fake boobs, removing ribs for that tiny waist. Not many other cultures in the world apart from North America have this problem quite so bad. If you've done some traveling, you've probably already realized this. The media has brainwashed us into believing this is the ideal body we should strive for. It also means that unfortunately, in some arenas, more success will come your way in North America if you fit these ideals. It hasn't always been this way certainly. Take a look back to the 1950s, when the voluptuous hourglass figure was 'in'. Super-sexy Marilyn Monroe wore a size 14 and every woman wanted her figure; today a size 14 is considered a plus size! You sure won't find a size-14 actress playing the lead/love-interest in any blockbuster film these days. The average movie star is below a size zero, and shrinking rapidly! So just how did we get so screwed up over time and where will all this lead? It can be very hard to tune out the media and what they're telling us we need to be and start listening to our own voices. These ideas may give you a place to start muffling those messages:

- Visit other countries who admire big butts, curvy hips, muscular legs, and voluptuous breasts. Try South America, the Middle East, India, or the Caribbean.
- If you can't travel, hang out with people from other parts of the world. You'll be surrounded by folks with very different thoughts on what a beautiful body is.
- Take bellydance – it embraces a woman's body, a woman's curves. It's a myth that you need to have a big belly to bellydance. This art form is beautiful on all women's bodies.
- Take up power lifting. Or Taekwondo. Or swimming. Or any sport where strong muscular form is valued as beautiful.
- Think back to when you truly felt beautiful, powerful, fit, or sexy? What were you doing? Who were you with? Recapture that time.

Your Personal Dream Body

Now that we've dismissed the idea that your automatic ideal body doesn't need to be stick thin, it's time to decide exactly how you DO want to look. Next is assessing how realistic that body goal is in relation to what you're willing to do to get it. This is the fun part... so get excited!

Your first assignment is to flip through magazines, surf websites, look at photos (maybe even past photos of yourself), and find a few images of how you might like your body to look. Keep these photos where you can see them all the time – maybe on the fridge, your mirror, your journal or calendar. You could put one in each place. People are often surprised when they visit my house to find clippings of sexy ladies in bikinis all over the place, but what can I say - it works for me! These pics are terrific inspiration and can rev you up and keep you motivated as you face your daily challenges.

Do you want...
- an athletic toned physique?
- a more curvy feminine figure?
- just to lose those last five pounds?
- or do you still want that super-slim look? (that's fine as long as YOU really want it for yourSELF, to make YOU happy)

Whatever you decide you really want for you and not just to fit into a certain mold, you can make it happen! You now need to decide how important it is for you to look this way: Is it more important than enjoying that daily chocolate bar? Is it more important than sleeping in every morning and missing your workout? Is it more important than indulging in after-work drinks a few times a week?

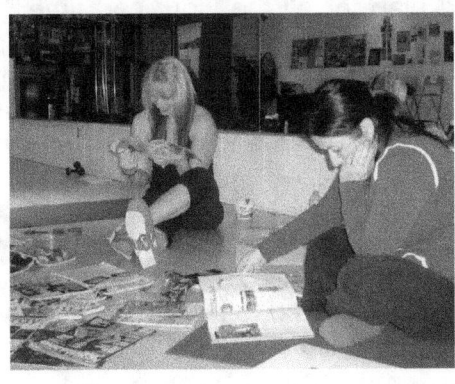

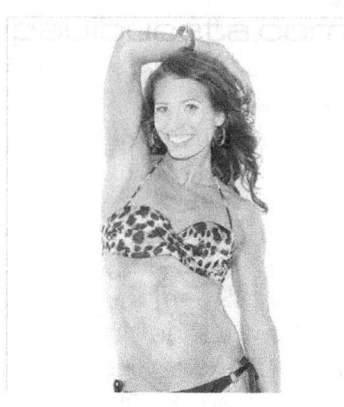

No answer is right or wrong – it's all about priorities. You might decide that eating those chocolate bars is something you're not willing to give up to lose those last lose ten pounds. Just make sure that you are really happy about what you're doing and not fibbing to yourself. Usually you can find a compromise like cutting your chocolate intake in half and not losing quite as much weight. And it's vital to realize that those hot bods you see on TV, in movies, or in magazines are the result incredibly strict eating regimens coupled with hours of grueling workouts every day. Keeping bodies looking great is part and parcel of the job if you're a model or film actor. Many of you will have other jobs that aren't quite as dependent on how you look in a bikini. So really think about how much time, energy, and commitments you're willing and able to make. Remember that the more extreme a change you want to make (for example, if you're extremely overweight and long to be a Kate Moss look-alike) – the more extreme your plan will have to be. I'm definitely not saying you shouldn't dream big – I believe you should in every aspect of your life! But you do need to consider, acknowledge, and plan for all the work and time it will take you to get to your big goal. If you're too unrealistic and think it will be a breeze, you'll quickly run into disappointment. So if you want a big dramatic body change – brace yourself for a big dramatic change in your lifestyle and what you can and can't do! As with most things in life, you reap what you sow.

Now I bet some of you are thinking "But my friend Suzy eats everything in sight, never exercises, and has such a great slim body! I guess I'm just destined to be fat... it's in my genes... I have a slow metabolism... nothing will help me – it's not fair!" No, it isn't fair – it really isn't. But it is life. So stop the blame-game and realize you may have to work harder than skinny Suzy to get and keep weight off. Realize also that the grass is always greener on the other side... Skinny Suzy may be so prone to being underweight that she's working hard to put weight ON. Oh I know anyone who has over-weight issues really doesn't like to hear this, but I've known and worked with many skinny women who would give just about anything to have a more curvy feminine figure. My grandma, who had that tall slender build that most women in our culture envy, was always telling me she wanted to be fatter! She pointed out pictures of little old ladies who were round and pudgy and would say "I wish I could look cute like this!" Most overweight people can't understand how much these naturally lean people want to gain weight. It can be just as hard, or even harder, for these types to gain weight as it is for us to take it off. I give naturally skinny people looking to gain weight just about the same advice I give everyone else... if it means a lot to you to change your body, you'll need to work hard at it whether it's losing or gaining weight. If you don't CARE enough to DO enough that's okay; just don't whine and complain when you could be fixing the 'problem'. You just don't want it enough at this particular time. So next time you see a skinny gal chowing down heartily, stuffing her face at every opportunity, don't be jealous – she may be working on her goals just like you are!

Action Plan:
- *Explore different beauty ideals*
- *Decide what you truly want your body to look like and collect/post inspiring images*
- *Decide how badly you want it*
- *Realize this journey will not be the same for everyone*

SETTING GOALS

Now that you have an idea of what you really want, let's get busy setting some real achievable, but also super-exciting, goals. These will keep you going strong through your journey!

When setting goals, we're often told to be realistic. I want to encourage you to forget that and reach for the stars! Stop holding yourself back by being too realistic about everything. Get dreaming big time and figure out what you really want for your body and your life in general. I'm not suggesting you set an impossible or unhealthy goal like losing thirty pound in a month or maintaining 2% body fat. I just want to invite you to smash your limiting beliefs and know that you can and will do anything you set your mind to!

Writing all your excuses or limiting beliefs down, then turning them around to become positive life-changing affirmations can be a super-powerful tool. What are your personal limiting beliefs? Sometimes you don't even realize the negative self-talk in your head. Start tuning into it and recording these falsehoods you tell yourself on a weekly, daily, or even hourly basis. For example, if you tell yourself something like "I love eating too much to lose weight", turn it around to "I am learning to love eating all sorts of new healthy foods that will make my weight loss dreams come true!"

Goal setting is one of the most important steps in making huge changes in your life. But it's very important not to just set a goal and then never look at it again. Our goals should become the basis of mantras that we will say over and over again to keep us on the right path. We will be setting short and a long term body-health goals as well as non-food rewards for staying on track.

Follow the SMART Goal Setting model
S = Specific
M = Measurable
A = Attainable
R = Realistic
T = Timely

Specific
You should be able to state clearly what you want to happen. Being very specific will keep your focus keen and help you to determine

what you need to do. So instead of saying you want to "lose weight" or "get healthy", it's more effective to set a more defined or specific goal like losing two inches off your waist measurement or exercising for 30 minutes a day. Think WHAT, WHY, and HOW.

WHAT are you going to do?

WHY is it important for you to do this at this time?

HOW will you accomplish it? (I'll do this by _____."

Measurable

You have to be able to track how things are going: how can you manage it if you can't measure it? Along the way to your big or overall goal, there are various smaller steps or successes that you'll be looking to accomplish as you progress. Identify the changes you'll be working to attain – be specific! – and give yourself target dates. "I want to lose weight and get in shape" is too vague and gives you no real, concrete criteria to measure your progress. If you decide, "I will lose five pounds by the end of the month, ten pounds by the end of next month, and twenty pounds before my beach vacation July 1st... you now have a timeframe to keep you on track. Each target date successfully reached will give you confidence and spur you onward!

Attainable

I know we talked about dreaming big, but you need to be aware and smart about this. If you set goals that are too far out of reach, you may feel overwhelmed and your commitment will falter. A goal should stretch you somewhat of course, so you feel you need to make a real push, a real commitment, to accomplish it. For instance, we all know that intending to lose twenty pounds in one week isn't achievable. But deciding to lose two pounds a week, and then when you've achieved that, working to lose a further two the next week, and then the next, is something you can do. And the feeling of success each week as you check off your goal will help keep you motivated. Have you heard of 'donut hole goals'? You know, donut holes are small, lovable, and easy to eat – kind of like little ambassadors of joy. That's an effective way to set goals: small, consumable goals on your way to your big goal!

Realistic

Please note that "realistic" is not the same as "easy". Realistic here simply means "do-able". That means do-able by YOU, where you are right now. Suppose you feel you need to give up your sugary, carby snack habit. You decide, "I'm swearing off chocolate bars, cake, fudge, cookies ... oh, and no more chips either! EVER. That's it!" If you're someone who really looks forward to and enjoys these little treats every day, how realistic do you think that never/ever/no more goal is? A more do-able approach might be to say you're going to substitute a piece of fruit for one of those snack items tomorrow. The next day, maybe make two better-snack-choice substitutions... and so on. Realistic suddenly translates to more attainable!

Timely
Decide on a timeframe for the goal. Whether it's for next week, a month from now, or two years down the road, attaching an end point to your goal gives you a clear target to work towards. Without a target date, it's easy for commitment to waver. Why is that? Simply because you feel you can start getting serious any time - there's no urgency to start taking action NOW.

Keeping all this new goal-setting wisdom in mind, your assignment now is to set at least three short-term goals – things you want to achieve in the next three months. I want one of these to be measurement-based (losing 10 pounds, losing 3 inches off your hips, going down a dress size), one should be feeling-based (loving workouts, jumping out of bed with tons of energy, being happy to look in the mirror and really admiring your reflection), and one should be event-based (running a 5K in less than 30 minutes, rocking a hot dress at your office party, feeling great in your bikini on your upcoming vacation to Cuba). Its not enough to just sit there and think of goals... stop reading now and write those goals down! NOW! Its also not enough to write them down and never look at them again... Post them around your house, in your wallet, anywhere you'll see them throughout the day. Read them aloud daily to remind yourself of what you're working to achieve. If you want to set more than three, go for it... have fun!

Action Plan:
- *Write your limiting beliefs down, turn them around to become positive affirmations*
- *Write down at least three SMART goals – measurement, feeling. and event based*
- *Post your goals where you're sure to see them throughout the day*
- *Read your goals out loud at least once a day*

IT ALL STARTS WITH LOVE

From Within

You are more than your body and how you look. And my wish – my mission! – is for you to get to a place where you can see that. It's important for you to recognize and appreciate all the good that's inside: are you funny? kind? strong? resilient? Start by grabbing your journal and writing down as many words as you can think of that describe your personality. Don't just take a shortcut here and think of a few in your mind – I want you to WRITE THEM DOWN. If this is hard for you to do on your own, ask a few close friends or family members for some input to get the ball rolling.

And On the Outside: Your Sexy Reflection!

Okay, right now... take a moment, lift your top up, pull your pant legs up, or better yet get totally undressed and look into a full-length mirror. Really study yourself from all angles. What do you see? How do you feel? Does your reflection make you smile or are you full of hatred for all your perceived imperfections?

Here's an assignment: I want you to look at yourself in the mirror every morning, really taking everything in. Feel gratitude for your body. Find a few things you love about it and tell yourself – for example no matter what size I am my legs are super strong and athletic looking and I find that sexy. You may want to lose a lot of weight. You may want to tone up some areas, you may think you hate how your entire body looks right now, but I want you to really check yourself out and find some beauty that you can really admire and get excited about. If you're having trouble with this, pretend you're looking at someone else who might not have much body confidence. Tell them (you) about the positives, the beauty, you see.

Throughout your weight-loss journey you may start feeling better about your body and its different features, so it can be really fun to check out your progress every morning and celebrate what you've accomplished! But even more important than getting to your ideal body, and what will keep you doing what you need to do to get there is enjoying the process, congratulating yourself on small changes as you go, and having fun seeing your body at different stages of the journey. Nothing good will ever come from hate, it's as simple as that. Many weight-loss plans emphasize shame and body hatred to push you on to your big end goal. I believe if this is how you operate through a plan, you'll never be happy, and even when you lose all the pounds you planned to lose, you will nit-pick and find more to feel bad about. And you won't ever enjoy your body. I know people with the enviable body of a fitness model and the face of a super-model who still think they're ugly or fat. That's just crazy... and sad. And that's why it's crucial to make sure you find love for your body and appearance BEFORE you start this journey. I'm not suggesting there can't be things you want to change, but get the love going now, and watch it develop further and further as you go!

I've personally tried out almost every type of body, from chubby in my teenage years, to super fit and lean as a fitness competitor, to a more 'typical' or 'regular' body, to pregnant, to super overweight after being pregnant, and back through them all, a few times! I truly find the good in every look. When I'm holding onto a bit of fat, I embrace my curves and marvel at the fact I have boobs and a butt! When I'm super-lean, I enjoy showing off my toned abs and arms! When I'm pregnant I feel like a goddess because I'm creating a human being inside me! Of course I have my favorite look (which is somewhere in the middle), but I really never *hate* myself when I look in the mirror or see myself in pictures. I think there are two things that help me love myself at all stages: first, I've tried so many different looks so often in my life that I realize it's very fluid and can change at any moment depending where my focus is, and second, I know that I can fairly rapidly change my body one way or the other and I know just how to do it – what works for me. Many people get upset if they gain five or ten pounds or don't look like they did back in high school; I think this has a lot to do with not believing they can actually deal with it and make lasting changes. We will start by loving, loving, loving - and follow that up with KNOWING we can do this!

Selfies
I know, I know, people love to hate selfies. I personally love selfies, both public (on instagram or facebook) as well as private (just for me). I think when someone posts a selfie it's a beautiful thing. There is some thinking that people who post selfies are insecure and need validation; I actually believe it's quite the opposite. It says to me that the poster felt at their best at that moment and wanted to

celebrate that and share it with their online friends. I look at selfies as celebrations of life and of yourself! My IG & FB are unapologetically full of selfies, but I also take many private selfies, for my eyes only. At least once a week, sometimes daily, I like to do a quick mirror-selfie to see what's going on with my body. It helps me see what's good and what needs improvement. It allows me to confirm changes and check out progress. And looking at my body in a photo lets me see things more objectively than I can if I just look in the mirror. Why not grab your phone or ipad and start this plan with a selfie right now?

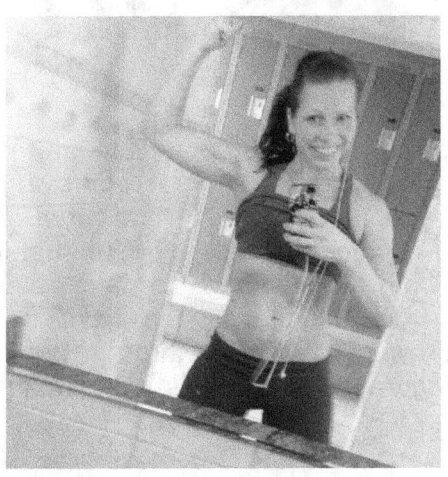

Don't Hate, Congratulate!

Get the love flowing to yourself by showing love to others! Appreciating others and yourself really do go hand in hand. Be generous with compliments to others as well as yourself. Someone else's super-fit bikini bod, disciplined eating habits, or successful completion of a marathon in no way detract from what you can do. In fact, they're points of inspiration: know that there's enough positives and success to go around... so get in the habit of appreciating, appreciating, appreciating!

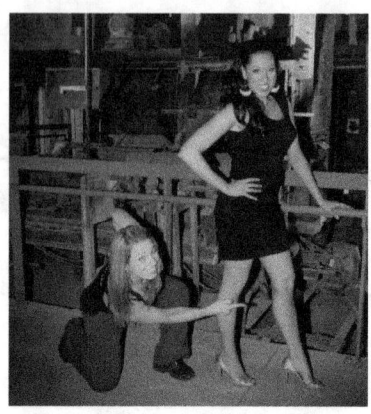

Loving Yourself Through the Process

I totally believe you can love and appreciate your body fully, while at the same time continuing to work at improving it. There's no disconnect here: you don't have to hate what you have to want something better. I came across a quote that I love: "You are allowed to be both a masterpiece and a work-in-progress, simultaneously." Simultaneously, at the same time, YES! Continuously improving your body through nourishing foods and enjoyable and invigorating exercise is actually an amazing form of love you can show your body. It's a gift – a luxury - you can give yourself.

I sometimes hear people talking about how much they love their curves or their big butt, saying that people tell them they look unwell if they lose weight. Now I am super happy for people who truly love their bodies, but sometimes I think people hide behind statements like these. This is especially true if they've always looked a certain way and they don't even know how they'd feel if they were healthier. Notice I say healthier, and not slimmer. Because the goal of being healthy really should trump the goal of being just slim. These kinds of statements also protect people from ever having to take action or make a change. Make sure you're not hiding behind some kind of 'fake' body-love. Love your body, cherish its uniqueness, appreciate the many things it does for you, and love the expedition to all that's possible that your body's on.

The time to get the love started is NOW! People often put off buying new clothes, going on vacation, dating, etc., until they reach their goal body or weight. This is the worst idea, really counterproductive. Giving yourself the love you need along the way will make you feel worth all the effort you're making on the way to your goal. I know, I know... you don't want to buy more plus-sized clothes because then it makes you feel like you're going to be staying there, right? But think about how terrific a new dress could make you feel during this process. And remember you can always buy another dress in another size in a month or two... won't that be exciting! If money is an issue, buy second-hand or less expensive clothing for your temporary sizes. Just do not walk around hating your reflection in the mirror because you refuse to buy clothing until you get to the end. This is a waste of life! Your life doesn't begin when you become a size 6! The same goes for getting your hair done or springing for that cool gel mani-pedi. It's even more important to do these things along the way as a way to say "I love you" to yourself!

Action Plan

- *Write down and celebrate all your awesome personality traits*
- *Check out your beautiful reflection and praise your amazing body daily*
- *Take mirror selfies*
- *Appreciate and be inspired by other people's success*
- *Treat yourself throughout your journey, not only when you reach your goal*

GUIDELINES FOR EATING AND WORKING OUT

As already outlined, most of this book is focused on the mental roadblocks that can keep us from reaching our goals of managing our weight and getting fit. Of course there are some practical basics that have to be laid out, things like what to eat, when to eat, whether supplements are required, and what exercises your workout should include.

Many people look at losing weight as a simple equation: less calories in, more calories out. Well, makes sense, right? People tend to translate that into "Oh no, I guess I'll just deprive myself of food (less calories in), and do hours and hours of boring cardio (more calories out)." And this is how they set themselves up for yet another fat-loss failure.

Let's create a new paradigm! I'm going to spend just one chapter here on the basics you need for fat-blasting eating and exercise. It's not going to be specific or mathematical, it's going to be general and fairly common sense. But listen up... because from these basics you'll learn how your body responds and you can adjust as you go. The results you're ultimately after await – let's go!

How to Eat
I recommend that you eat somewhere from 1500 - 2000 calories a day to start losing weight depending on your size, activity level, etc. People often feel to eat so low-calorie, you need to eat less. The reality is that you don't need to change the quantity of what you eat, as much as the quality. Most clients tell me that they feel weight-loss meal plans I create for them are super-filling and that there's actually too much food! When you eat the way we are going to be eating here, you'll be eating a lot and may even find it challenging to take in enough calories each day.

Eat five small meals a day, starting as soon as you wake up and spread evenly throughout your day. Each meal should be approximately 300 - 400 calories. Combine a healthy carb and a lean protein from the lists below, including some healthy fats along the way. Here are just a few examples:

HEALTHY CARBS	LEAN PROTEINS	BENEFICIAL FATS
Fruits	skinless chicken breast	coconut oil
Greens	lean ground turkey	Nuts
brown rice	Fish	natural nut butters
sweet potato	eggs/egg whites	Avocado
slow cooked oats	cottage cheese	olive oil

Example of a day of healthy eating:

7:00am	1 egg with ½ cup egg whites & slow cooked oats with raisins & cinnamon
11:00am	1 cup low-fat cottage cheese with berries
2:00pm	4 oz salmon, 8 asparagus spears, 1 cup brown rice
5:00pm	10 almonds & 1 apple
8:30pm	4 oz skinless chicken breast, small sweet potato, 1 cup broccoli

How to Workout

You will read later about how to find workouts you'll love and look forward to, but right now all I'm going to say is start with 30 minutes of sweaty movement each day. You could do a gym workout, an at-home workout, an outdoor workout, or different stuff each day to keep you interested. Below I have outlined a very basic idea of a workout you can do at home in case you need an actual idea:

20 minutes cardio (brisk walking, jogging, or running around your area or on a treadmill, skipping, jumping around to music, whatever gets you sweaty!)
20 minutes of strength training (no equipment necessary: push-ups, sit-ups, planks, squats, lunges, step-ups, etc.)

Action Plan
- *Eat 5 small meals of 300 – 400 calories each, made up of lean protein,*
  healthy carb, and some good fat. Eat about every 3 hours
- *Get sweaty for at least 30 minutes each day*

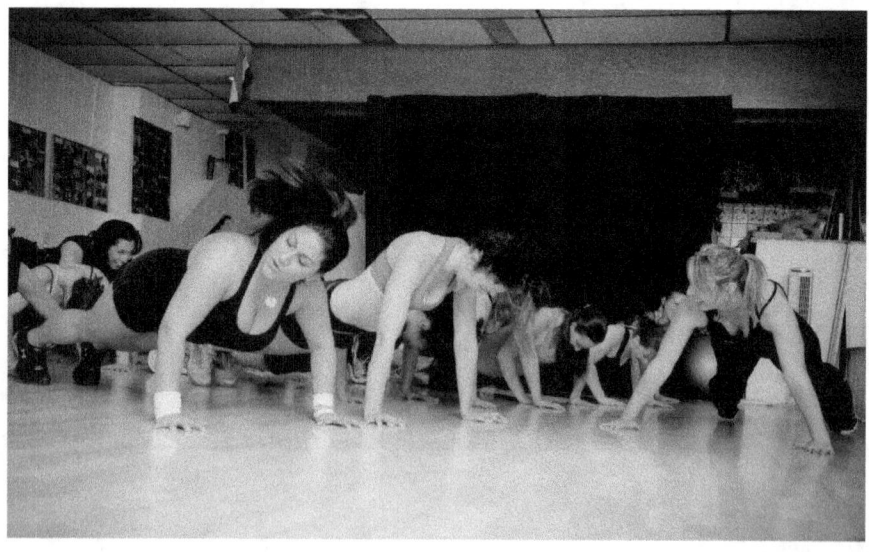

LOVING HEALTHY FOODS

What you eat, more than anything else, will determine how your body will look and how you will feel. I believe how you look is about 80% what you eat, and 20% genetics and exercise. THIS IS SOMETHING YOU NEED TO UNDERSTAND AND ACCEPT FOR SUCCESS. PERIOD. Of course I also believe what you eat will be greatly affected by many of the points in this book, things like whether you had a great workout to start your day, whether you're feeling in love with yourself and your life, the people you're surrounding yourself with, etc. Until you figure out all the stuff in your head, eating clean will likely be a struggle and achieving your ultimate fitness will be difficult.

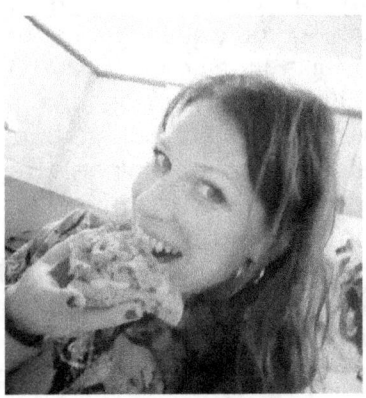

Let's take a look at the three types of people when it comes to eating healthy. See where you might fit in… and what you can do to modify or tone up your approach!

First there are the people who *think* they don't like healthy foods. They rarely eat them or only eat them when they 'have' to to look good for a certain event or occasion. These people would benefit from being a little more open-minded and having a good attitude about trying all sorts of new foods. I've had so many people tell me they hate egg whites, cottage cheese, oatmeal, and other fabulously healthy foods that could help them achieve their goals. I always suggest first of all that they try different spices and stuff that change the taste of these foods a bit to see if that helps. I let them know that what works for me is tons of cinnamon in my oatmeal, hot sauce on my egg whites, and fruit in my cottage cheese. People often think eating clean has to be drab and boring like plain chicken breast with broccoli. I want you to go crazy and cook up some amazing garlic/ginger chicken stir-fry with tons of beautiful vegetables! Get excited about trying new foods and spices. You will never feel beautiful while eating bland boring foods you hate! Learn to love new healthy foods! Don't look at eating healthy foods as punishment, look at it as a luxury for your body and delicious fuel for your engine, the very best way to celebrate YOU!

Next we have the people who *think* they are eating healthy consistently and wonder why it's not working for them. In most cases, anyone truly eating the right proportions of super-healthy foods 90% of the time can't help but look fairly fit. That's it. So if you haven't reached your goal even though you think you're eating well, try writing everything you eat down in a food journal. Or record it in an app or website like fitday.com or My Fitness Pal. You need to record EVERYTHING. Every single thing. Don't conveniently 'forget' to note down snacks like chocolate bars, lattes, bites of your kid's leftovers, or that late-night chip binge! Be brutally honest here - only you will see this. Often we trick ourselves into thinking we are being so healthy, but there are all sorts of extras we *forget* about. When you record it all, you start to see the true picture. A little education can also be helpful, as many items that people tend to think of as healthy are often not the best choices. These include things like whole grain bread made with belly-bloating gluten or protein bars full of sugar.

Then there are the people who actually eat healthy most of the time. These people may be fortunate enough to just naturally prefer food and portions that are good for their bodies, or they may work hard to manage their nutrition. If you eat healthy and you're feeling great (and are sure you're not fooling yourself with what category YOU fall into), you probably don't have any food issues and can skip or dance or somersault your way on to the next section!

Action Plan
- *Realize that how you eat is the biggest factor that determines how you look and feel*
- *Figure out what your roadblock is to clean eating and take steps to remedy it*

EXERCISE: YOUR BEST FRIEND

Sweat for 30 - 60 minutes each day. It's that easy! You read this prescription in the last chapter; as long as you're working it hard for at least 30 minutes a day - and loving it! - you're good. Of course if you have specific areas you want to tone or curves you want to accentuate, weight training is awesome. Working out with weights also has a host of other benefits like turning fat into muscle and speeding up your metabolism/burning more calories at rest. Cardio is great for fat-burning, heart-helping, and mood-enhancing. So why wouldn't you cover all bases and combine weight-training and cardio?

Lovin' It!
I absolutely LOVE exercise!!! I know you're probably rolling your eyes and groaning right about now. Being a personal trainer, the most common things I hear are, "I just hate to exercise", "Exercise is boring", "I just can't make myself do it", and "I don't have time to exercise". I believe this is because most people have a very narrow-minded idea of what exercise is. Often what springs to mind is hours of monotonous cardio on a machine at a gym, like a gerbil in its wheel. I'm here to tell you, that is not what I want you to do or feel towards exercise. I don't want it to be a necessary evil, I want it to be what gets you going, what makes you feel alive, what can snap you out of a bad mood in minutes! I want it to be an integral part of your day, something you might even look forward to!

Think back to what physical activity you loved as a child or teenager. It doesn't have to be a sport, I was the furthest from a sporty child or teen; for me, it was all about dance. Dancing is still my passion! What was your thing? Judo... skipping... soccer... swimming... hula-hooping? This is often a good place to start. And if you weren't a particularly active child, no worries – just stay open-minded about all that there is to try. Think about all the choices out there and pick an active form of play to engage in each and every day for at least thirty minutes. You can start small and work up to an hour a day.

It's easy to forget many great things about exercise! Exercise creates feel-good hormones called endorphins, so even if at first it doesn't seem like much fun, you will get addicted to the after-effect of exercise. My mood can definitely suffer if I miss a few days of working out. I believe anyone who doesn't exercise regularly is pretty much always in this state, they just don't realize it. I believe anti-anxiety and anti-depressant drugs would go out of business if more people would just exercise and love it everyday! Try it for a month – do something you love physically every day and marvel at how you feel! Apart from all this inner good exercise can do, of course there's a whole world of outer good too. This is where you may want to get more focused and integrate some weight training. Weight training is something women often shy away from because they "don't want to look like a man". Let's dispel this myth. You will rarely end up looking masculine with tons of huge muscles unless you take steroids, work for years, and eat a whole whack of calories! Women don't have the ability to become super-muscular unless they are doing something unnatural and hardcore. Some weight training a few times a week will help you lose fat and gain some muscle in all the right places – a round apple bottom, sexy feminine back, long and strong legs, and toned arms. If you only do cardio and diet, you can become what is called 'skinny-fat' and you will still be complaining about your loose skin, overhangs, and jiggles. Instead, of course you want to be sexy, tight, and toned – so pick up those weights!

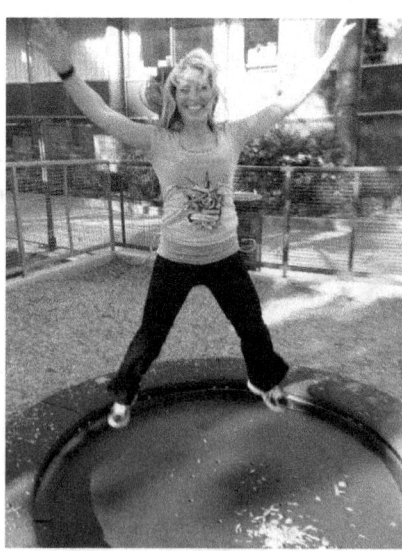 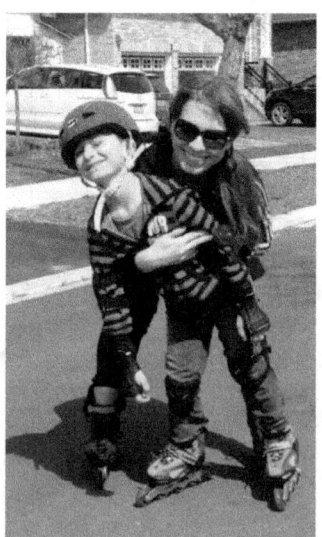

Making Time for Exercise

Ah, the notorious time issue. Aren't you worth that one hour or less that you're going to commit to yourself and your fitness? YES, YOU ARE. It's hard to believe how many people put watching TV's "The Bachelor" or surfing Facebook or Pinterest way ahead of their own well-being. Put down the remote control, set your alarm an hour earlier, or tell your family that you need to go to the gym while they're watching Netflix. Whatever it takes, just do it, carve out that time. Start looking at it as a privilege, not a punishment! You are enriching your mind, soul, and body inside and out when you exercise and you love it. Have a great open positive attitude towards all the exercise you do. Figure out what you love most, what makes you feel great, and what time works best for exercise. Is it:

- An outdoor jog or rollerblade early in the evening?
- A rocking upbeat dance-exercise class at the rec center after work?
- Cardio & weight training at the gym as you start your day?
- Getting together with friends or co-workers for a game of soccer or floor hockey?

Whatever it is, make it a habit. You're more likely to get on a regular schedule of working out and stick to it if you make it a habit and commit to a regular time each day or during the week. You might decide to sign up for a workout class at the local community center or gym every Monday, Wednesday, and Friday at 6:30pm, for instance. Or try what I find the best habit to get into, especially if you're super-busy with family and work life and everything else you do: get up each weekday before everyone else and get your gym workout in before the day starts. This is like magic and really sets you up for a healthy and happy day! Whatever you think is going to work best for you and your schedule - do it. Plan your workouts and when they'll happen, then make sure to keep this important appointment with yourself. The last person in the world you should flake out on is you!

Action Plan
Figure out what type of exercise is going to excite you and do that
Carve out the time to workout and make it a habit

HABITS

As Albert Einstein said, "Insanity is doing the same thing over and over again and expecting different results." You've probably already tried various diets, exercise regimes, and strategies, but you're reading this because you're still looking for something. You may be surprised at what I want you to do next... try more! Keep an open-mind and try some other ideas to see what will work best for you, your goals, and your lifestyle. Following are two habits I want you to consider trying...

Eating the same thing every day
I've been a nutrition counsellor for years and when people come to me initially for a meal plan, I usually put them on a very simple plan made up of 4 – 6 small meals a day - lean protein, greens, with a few healthy carbs and fats in a few of the meals. I instruct them to eat the same menu each day. At first, new clients think this will be boring and I get a little resistance. They soon find, though, that the simplicity and habit-forming effect of this plan makes it super-useful for kick-starting their new healthy eating regimes. This way, there's no room for wondering what to snack on or for creatively justifying substituting pizza for your chicken and broccoli. You know what you need to eat and when and you need to do it; there's no grey area where you're left trying to decide if you should do something else or if you could have that cheeseburger on your way home from work. It also gets you into the practice of eating specific things at regular intervals and creates... that useful habit! In addition, it makes meal prep easier as you know exactly what you eat each day and can prep in bulk for the week.

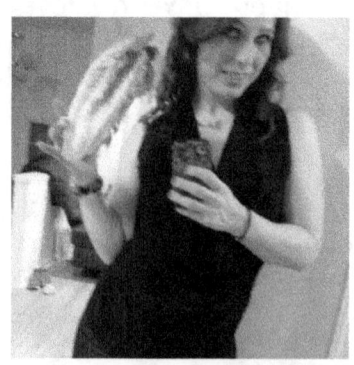

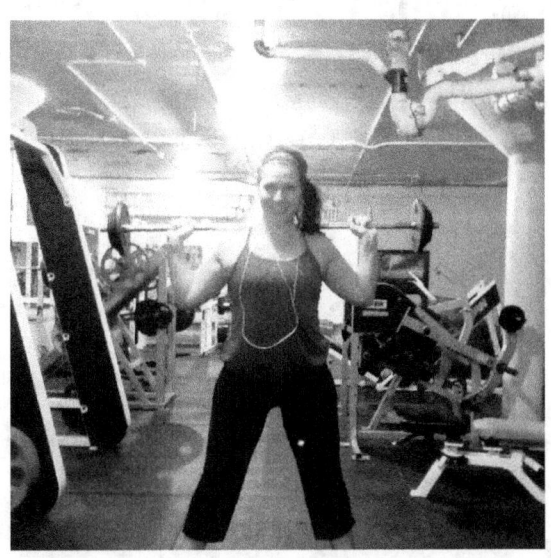

Working out at the same time every day
The specific time you choose is less important than deciding you will set aside that time and work out then every day. I highly recommend waking up early and getting your sweat on before the rest of your day starts. I find this the most effective especially with a busy life, family, work, and all the other demands on your time. You guarantee you'll get your workout in, you start your day off right, and you don't have to worry about procrastinating or maybe missing it entirely when your day gets too hectic or difficult. If early morning's not possible for you, find another time like right after work, on your lunch hour, in the afternoon while your baby sleeps, or late-night. Just allot a certain time for your workout and stick to it. It will soon become a habit and a refreshing, renewing time you'll look forward to!

Action Plan
- *Experiment with eating the same thing every day and working out at the same every day to see if it's for you*

FINE-TUNING YOUR ENVIRONMENT FOR SUCCESS

Time to give some thought to several other things that you need to manage so they don't hold you back on the way to your fitness goals.

Toxic People
Most people who doubt you, put you down, or make fun of your get-fit efforts may not actually mean to. They may be fighting many of their own limiting beliefs and problems that they end up projecting them onto you. It may be painful to them to see you working towards all your goals when they aren't. Remember that you can do anything you set your mind to regardless of what others think or say; it's what you think and say to yourself that matters. Rather than letting the naysayers bring you down, think about trying to help them realize their goals and dreams. They may not be as ready as you are this point in time, and that's okay too. Sometimes, though, you may need to cut ties with certain people if their negativity is too infectious. Surrounding yourself with people who support and celebrate your new path will give you a boost.

Limiting Thoughts
You need to believe that anything is possible! Let's look at how brainwashing can work against you… or FOR you:

You've probably been thinking one way for your entire life. Now if you're going to make big lifestyle and mental changes, you really need to brainwash yourself to stay in this mode and keep you from slipping back to your old less healthy and perhaps self-doubting ways. We're always being warned about the dangers of brainwashing, but let's look at it in a different way and harness its power for GOOD! I like to think of brainwashing as actually 'washing' the brain – cleaning it out and replacing the old, dusty, 'broken' ideas with new shiny ones.

Ways to brainwash yourself:
-   Post inspirational pictures, goals, and quotes on your fridge, at your desk at work, in your wallet, etc. to keep you in the right mindset. Look at them when you're wavering. An even better and stronger idea is to make a vision board – a collage you create by pasting newspaper/ magazine/

computer print-off clippings onto a board or in a frame. Hang it in a prominent spot where you'll see it every day. Let it remind you of what you're working towards. You can also make a vision board online and keep it as your desktop and phone wallpaper.

- Read health and fitness magazines and books, watch fitness television shows like "the Biggest Loser", "X-weighted", "Last 10 pounds Boot Camp"". These will help educate you and keep you in the healthy lifestyle world.

- Check out internet sites regularly for new healthy recipes, forums, exercises, and articles. Follow a favorite fitness blogger (or maybe even think about starting a blog yourself!) These things will help keep you super inspired.

- Incorporate some powerful mantras into your day. Make these simple, direct, and super-positive. Repeating "I will rock that mini-dress at the holiday party" or "I enjoy eating new healthy foods that enrich my body inside and out", can really keep your mind in the game. Make it second nature to repeat these while working out, grocery shopping, walking to the store.

- Most of all, take time every day to show yourself the love you so deserve and enjoy your beautiful body every step of the way.

Accountability

Try recording everything you eat in a journal and/or on a handy and educational app like myfitnesspal or fitday.com. You can learn so much about your eating habits, why you eat certain things when you shouldn't (for example eating a big slice pizza that wasn't on your plan because you went all day without eating). It's also very inspiring and useful to record your workouts, either in a notebook in lots of detail or something as little as a happy face on a calendar to confirm you worked out. Weigh yourself, take measurements, and record results at the start of this new journey, and each week as you go to track progress and figure out if any changes need to be made. As much as this can be a little scary or weird, I strongly suggest you tell friends, family, people you're close with at work about your goals (even big, hard to imagine ones!). Putting it out there, making it 'public' in this way can be a big motivator, holding you accountable and challenging you to follow through. While all this outside accountability is helpful, you also need to hold yourself accountable to the most important person - YOU!

Groceries & Prep

I recommend making a list and grocery shopping once a week for all the staples. Then you can grab fresh fruit and veggies throughout the week. The idea is to have lots of healthy options in your fridge and cupboards at all times, ready to go when you're hungry. The same goes for when you're out and about: prepare a full day's worth of meals and snacks and pack it in a cooler so you never get stuck anywhere without your healthy meals. Streamline your prep and make your life easier by preparing your food for a few days in advance. You can clean and cut veggies and fruit, measure out single servings of cottage cheese and yogurt, seal things in containers, cook meat and eggs, etc.

Socializing

Don't think that you have to lock yourself up and become a hermit throughout this process to avoid things like alcohol and munchies! Remember that the idea is to create eating and lifestyle changes that you can and will continue forever. A balanced lifestyle means you can indulge in a piece of cake at a party and not feel bad or guilty about it. I recommend having one cheat meal a week when you can eat (and drink) anything you want. Try to schedule this meal for when you know there's a social event you'll be attending so you can really let loose, have a drink and some yummy food. If you happen to be a social butterfly and go out a few times a week, just choose salad with grilled chicken, or fish and steamed veggies. Every restaurant has something healthy you can eat. Try to stay positive about this process rather than complaining about what you can't have.

Support

Although this is a very personal journey you're on, I highly recommend finding a buddy to 'travel' with. Make sure your buddy is on the same page as you, has read this book, and is just as ready as you are to make a new start. This could be your partner, a friend, a family member, or even an online friend. It's great if you can work out and perhaps prepare food together, as well as monitor (and celebrate) each other's progress, but it could also be someone who you check in with once a day or once a week, and discuss challenges, feelings, and achievements with. Whatever you decide on, make sure you have a regular set time to chat about things. Many people won't be able to relate to what you're going through, so it can be very helpful to have a connection with someone who will… because they're on the same path.

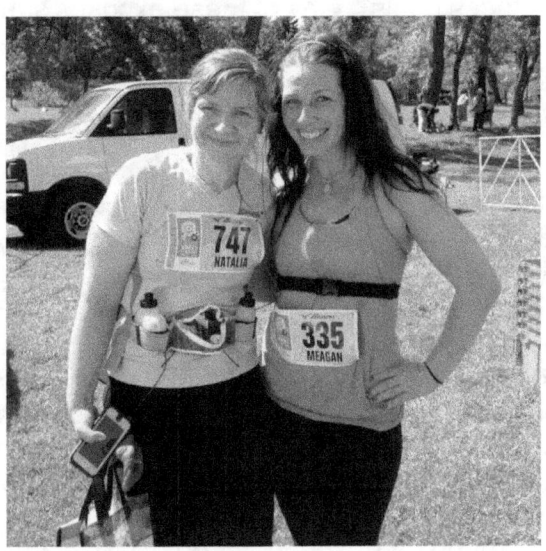

Action Plan
- *Rid your life of toxic people and limiting beliefs. Instead surround yourself with supportive people who spur you on*
- *Brainwash yourself into positivity with books, tv, inspirational posts, etc.*
- *Make a day when you do most of your groceries and prep food for the week*
- *Don't give up your social life, just tweak it. Remember your priorities when out on the town*
- *Get a support buddy*

OVERCOMING EXCUSES

Everyone's got 'em, but they sure won't help you in your quest to get fit or for doing anything else either! What justifications or 'reasons' do you tell yourself and others about why you aren't reaching your fitness goals? Any of these excuses sound familiar?

1) I would lose weight, BUT…
I eat when I'm depressed / lonely / bored, and I seem to be depressed / lonely / bored a lot.

If deep down inside you turn to unhealthy food for comfort, you need to take two very important steps. First, figure out why you're so depressed / lonely / bored and then, start making changes in your life to remedy this. If you're depressed (and it's not a doctor-diagnosed clinical depression), decide on steps to improve your life in the areas that are currently keeping you less than happy. You're reading this book, so it could be that your body and health is making you depressed; often it can be a vicious cycle of being depressed because you aren't happy with the way your body looks and feels, then you overeat because of that feeling and it just makes things worse, cycling 'round and 'round. Look into learning to soothe yourself with something other than food. Try socializing, exercising (sweating it out!), meditation, throwing yourself into a hobby you enjoy. Is it a different stressor/depressor you're living with? A relationship perhaps? Your career… or lack of? Are you lonely? Are you lacking passion in your life? Your job is to identify it and FIX it! Of course that's easier said than done, but it's important to figure this out and deal with it head-on. You don't, however, have to finish this up *before* you start your own love yourself fit journey. Do it all simultaneously, the two missions really do go together and will have many crossovers.

2) I would lose weight, BUT…
I just had a baby! I gained so much weight when I was pregnant and now I'm focused on my newborn and have no time to think about my own body.

Look around at women with babies. They all have different bodies – some are still carrying extra pregnancy weight, others are back to their pre-pregnancy selves, others have actually improved their bodies after having given birth. What does all this mean? Not all mothers stay large and round after giving birth - it's just like being a woman who hasn't had a child: you have a choice whether you have your ideal body or not. Certainly it may be harder because you're up all night trying to put your baby to sleep, and you're so busy worrying about this new child that you don't seem to have time to think about yourself or what you're eating. But that doesn't mean you should just give up and resign yourself to a life of looking like a frumpy mom. Don't you want to be a yummy-mummy like J. Lo or Beyonce? Look at celebrities who lose their baby fat in a few weeks for their next role in a movie. I'm not saying this is the way to go, it just shows that it can be done! And you will allot yourself a much more reasonable time frame for your post-baby weight loss so you do it in a healthful way. Do I hear another 'BUT' forming in your mind? Something about celebs having nannies, personal trainers, chefs, and all the time and money in the world so it's so easy for them? And how it's their job to look a certain way? All true, but imagine how awesome and invincible you can feel knowing you got your ideal bod through your own hard work, time management, knowledge, and sweat! Even with baby around, carve out some time for yourself. I'm not suggesting you abandon your family and go to the spa every day, just recommending you take an hour or so each day that's all yours. To think about what your priorities are, to go for a jog outside, get a massage, plan and prep your healthy meals for the coming week.

Post-baby, it's also just important to prioritize your health. How will you have the energy to keep up with your child if you're an overweight, lazy couch potato? And consider what type of example you're setting; a child who grows up never seeing you be active, eating Big Macs, and never making time for yourself, will pick up these bad habits, and potentially end up having to deal with the results of unhealthy living themselves. You don't want that to happen!

3) I would lose weight, BUT…
I'm addicted to sweets/fried food/chips/etc!

Many studies have shown that sweets and white flour products are very addictive substances. The more you eat, the more you crave. If you stop eating them cold turkey, you suffer withdrawal symptoms similar to people who quit smoking, drinking alcohol, or using recreational drugs. These addictions can be strong. I am a total sugar addict and probably always will be, so I totally understand how hard it can be to lose weight when you're so addicted to junk food. I can empathize, but know this isn't a valid excuse to let your body go! These are some ways of coping you can try:

- Phase out bad sweets. If you have dessert or a sweet treat after every meal, try eating desert after only one meal a day.
- Start replacing your bad sweets with more healthful sweets. Try substituting ice cream or a candy bar with fruit or yogurt topped with a bit of honey.
- My favorite: just go cold-turkey! Cut out all sweets and over-processed foods altogether. When your system's been free of all that nonsense for about two days, you'll find the cravings just... stop. Don't be all skeptical, give it a try!
- Educate yourself on the harm sugar and refined carbs can do to your body and mind. Watch documentaries, read books - there's a lot of info out there linking sugar to all kinds of ailments and terrible diseases. Having this knowledge can be a powerful tool in keeping these addictions under control.

4) I would lose weight, BUT...
My partner/family/people I'm around all the time eat unhealthy foods – temptation is there at every turn!

This can definitely be tough, but is definitely fixable! You either bring the person or persons along for the awesome healthy ride, or you get tough and resist the temptations! If it's someone you live with, try getting them on board so you only need to keep healthy foods in the house. I often hear from mothers that they're so tempted by their kids' treats... hey, you do the grocery shopping – DON'T BUY THAT STUFF! I'm not saying you should never let your kids eat cookies, cake, etc., just don't keep them on YOUR shelves or in YOUR fridge. Let them have a special treat when you're all at the movies or out for dinner. If your partner or other adults you live with aren't interested in changing their lifestyle with you, you'll just need to buckle down and resist! Can they keep their unhealthy items in a cupboard you never open so you're not faced with temptation all the time? Be resourceful, you can figure this out!

5) I would lose weight, BUT...
I have a medical problem that keeps me overweight.

Yes, many medical conditions and medications they require can make it more difficult to lose weight, some even make you gain weight. I personally have thyroid issues, but I like to think of it a little differently: instead of blaming my thyroid for making me not look and feel the way I ultimately want to, I think of it as even more of a reason to really eat right and get lots of exercise in. I try to think about how much worse my thyroid problems might be if I was eating too much, eating the wrong things, or if I didn't work out. Having any sort of medical condition that makes you more susceptible to weight gain gives you an even stronger reason to embrace a healthy lifestyle. And of course healthy eating and regular exercise can only benefit whatever condition your body is suffering from on the inside too. So it's win/win. Don't ever feel defeated by your condition, genetics, or anything else!

6) I would lose weight, BUT…
I'm a social being – I eat out with friends all the time/Lots of business lunches and dinners are part of my job.

These days, there are always healthy options when eating out in restaurants. It's a matter of making up your mind to order the right things and not just give into that plate of creamy pasta and the basket of sourdough bread. Scan the menu for healthy choices; order a salad with a chicken breast or a chicken or beef stir-fry with lots of veggies. Skip the bread, drinks, and desserts. As long as you don't make a federal case out of how it's so hard to eat healthy, how you'll miss those fries and gravy, people you're with won't be bothered. Decide before you walk into the restaurant that you'll stick with your healthy choices, then enjoy your meal, knowing it's bringing you closer and closer to your goal!

7) I would lose weight, BUT…
I'm too busy to prepare healthy meals or go to the gym.

If you've read this far, you probably know what I'm going to say… If it's truly important to you, you MAKE the time! Get up earlier, cut some of your TV time, multitask, do whatever it takes to make time for yourself. You are worth it. Life today is busy for everyone. Really think about what you're so busy WITH. Make sure the activities you choose to spend your time on are in line with, and bringing you closer to, your goals and dreams. Prioritize yourself!

8) I would lose weight, BUT…
I don't have enough money for nutritious foods / gym membership / personal trainer / etc.

It really doesn't have to cost anything! Of course having the luxury of a personal trainer to tell you what to do or a personal chef to cook all your healthy meals certainly would make it easier, do we really need easy? You're going to feel all the better achieving all your fitness goals if you did it yourself, plus you will learn so much as you go. Healthy foods don't have to cost a lot, oats, eggs, and tuna are some of the cheapest foods out there. Some fresh vegetables and cuts of meat and fish can sometimes be costly, but they don't need to always be on the menu. Also, think about the things you spend your money on now… fast food drive thrus? Happy Hour cocktails? Snacks of chips and candy throughout the day? Those are all going to be cut out in favor of clean healthy foods that you make and pack each day! As for workouts, there are tons of free ideas, you don't need a gym or a personal trainer, brisk walking or running is one of the best forms of cardio and all you need are some good supportive shoes! There are tons of at-home workout ideas that take very minimal or no equipment that you can find in books or online!

9)I would lose weight, BUT…
I'm intimidated by the gym.

For a newbie, certainly the idea of walking into a gym can be intimidating. The huge open space, filled with an array of mysterious and confusing machines, all the hardcore exercisers who seem like they're already in perfect shape – and who know what they're doing – can cause a quick "Oh, never mind". Signing up for the orientation that most gyms offer can help – a tour of the various areas and a demo of how the machines work will take the edge off any anxiety you may feel. You may find doing your gym workouts with a buddy puts you more at ease. Check out the local Y or recreation center for gyms with a somewhat more casual ambiance. Or buy a few weights and a skipping rope, add a workout video or two: instant home gym! Work out where you're comfortable… but work out!

Most excuses can be overcome by wanting your goal bad enough! Nothing else matters if you can really see that goal clearly and you want it badly enough. This is why it's super-important to keep your goals fresh in your mind and have reminders all the time of what you're working towards!

Action Plan
- *Figure out if you're using any of these excuses*
- *Focus on your goals rather than your excuses*

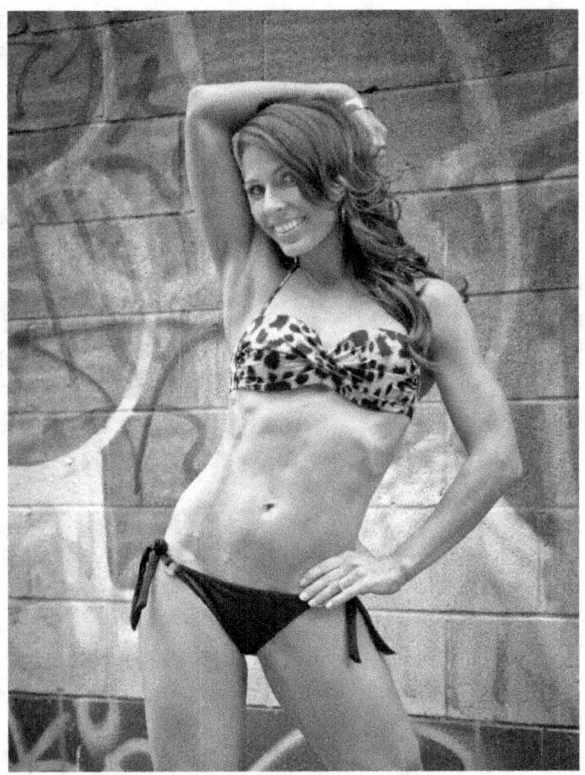

YOUR STARTING POINT

This is where it gets REAL! Take a photo of yourself in a bikini or underwear. Get good, clear front, back, and side views. Study the pictures and take notes on what parts you'd like to change. Do you aim to lose body fat all over? Tone your arms? Create less bulky – or more muscular! – legs? These notes are where you will start your goal-setting from. Take a moment, also, to write down what you like most about your body: is it your well-defined calf muscles, your slender waist, the shape of your breasts, your smile? Now put one of these shots up somewhere where you'll see it every day. (You might want to find a place where it's not easily seen by visitors or other people around – maybe inside your closet, you'll figure this out.) These photos can be quite the wake-up call: BE BRAVE – you need to know where you're starting from! And how exciting and empowering to know that you can move from where you are now to wherever you want to be - whether it's in your career, relationships, health, and of course how your body looks! As I mentioned before I also want you to celebrate this photo, think about what your body has done for you this far and what it will be doing for you in the future. Just because you want to make some changes, it doesn't mean you can't also love where you're at currently!

I also want you to weigh yourself and take measurements (upper arm, upper thigh, bust, waist, belly, hips) and record these as your starting point. I hear people defending their high weights all the time saying "Well, muscle weighs more than fat". This statement is very true, but if you lose some of the fat covering up all that muscle, your weight will go down! A 5'7" female fitness model may weigh 130 – 150 pounds, but no matter how much muscle she had, she probably wouldn't weigh 180 lbs. Or picture a huge male bodybuilder who is practically ALL muscle and only 5% body fat (which is insanely low). He might weigh in at 200 pounds... a whole body of that heavy muscle mass, and still he's under 200 lbs. And consider an unhealthy, overweight couch potato who has barely any lean muscle and tons of fat – they might weight upwards of 200 pounds... how the heck could they weigh so much if muscle weighs so much more than fat? These records of your weight and measurements are your jumping-off point – watch them change as your fitness story unfolds!

Its up to you how often you check your weight/measurements. Everyone is different, some people get discouraged by progress markers like weight, measurements, and photos, while it inspires others. Most plans tell you not to check progress too often or too soon, but sometimes I think It's great to check in every week or even more often so you can learn how your body works and how it reacts to different foods and workouts. I weigh myself every day just as an experiment and I think this can actually help you calm down and stop obsessing over what the scale says. For example, I don't freak out when the scale jumps up 4 pounds the day after indulging in pizza and ice cream... if I've been eating super-clean, my body gets shocked by junk and bloats up about 4 pounds, I know it's not permanent and that within a day or two, I will be back to my normal weight. Make sure you do weight, measurements, and photos as sometimes the weight won't budge, but you'll lose inches all over, or you'll notice dramatic differences in progress pics! Remember, weighing yourself can tell a story and can mark your progress sometimes, but inches and photos show the real picture of how your body looks, so please don't obsess about your weight not being a certain number! Whether it's recording progress every week, every month, or even less, figure out what type of time frame works for you personally and do that.

Action Plan
- *Take your starting point photo, weight, and measurements*
- *Figure out how often you will mark your progress and do it!*

CONCLUSION: NOW DO IT!!!

I hope you've had a good time reading this book, getting excited about your new life and body, and dreaming up some amazing goals you might not even have thought about before. Now make sure you take all this information and motivation and do something great with it! Too many times people read tons of advice, motivational stuff, etc. and then don't actually get off their butts and start working towards their goal... which was the reason they picked up the book in the first place! It's easy to read a book, it's fun to get excited by the motivation, but promise me you won't stop there. And you won't stop until you've achieved everything you want for your body and your life. Right now, start implementing the techniques we've talked about to start changing your mind, life, and body for the better. What will you do right now to start this journey? The journey to loving yourself fit! Make an action plan... and GO!

I'm so excited for your journey and encourage you to let me know how you are doing along the way. I want to hear your challenges, triumphs, achievements, everything!

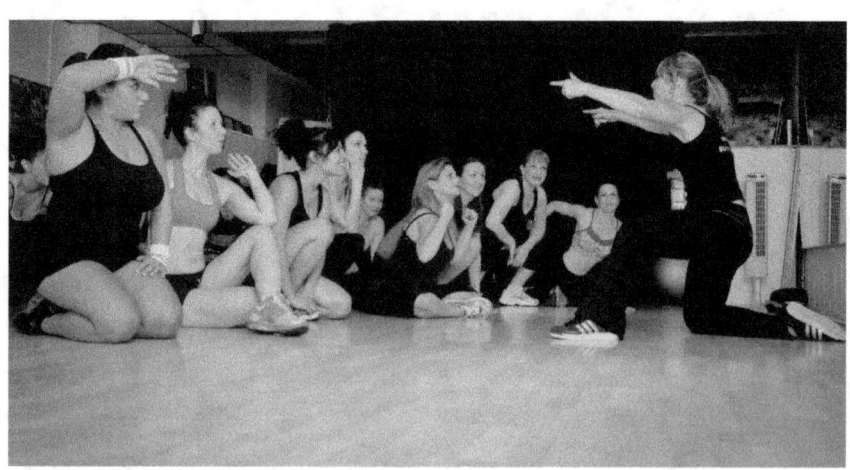

ACKNOWLEDGEMENTS

I would like to thank my mom for teaching me to always follow my heart, inspiring me to write, being an awesomely smart and strong role model, and listening to me blather on about my philosophies that ended up being this book.

Much love to my first bellydance instructor, Yasmina Ramzy who introduced me to the beautiful bellydance world and started my body image shift when I was a teenager. Also special thanks to all the amazing women I've met and worked with throughout my years in the dance and fitness world.

And this book would never have come to fruition without my soul mate, Walaa Hesham. Thanks for believing in me, supporting me, and showing me what love is all about!

CREDITS

Cover Photo Credit
Samira Hafezi

Cover Design
Pixelstudio

Interior Photo Credits
Samira Hafezi *(pages 4, 6)*
Natalia Sokolovska *(pages 6, 18, 22, 43)*
Paul Buceta *(page 10)*

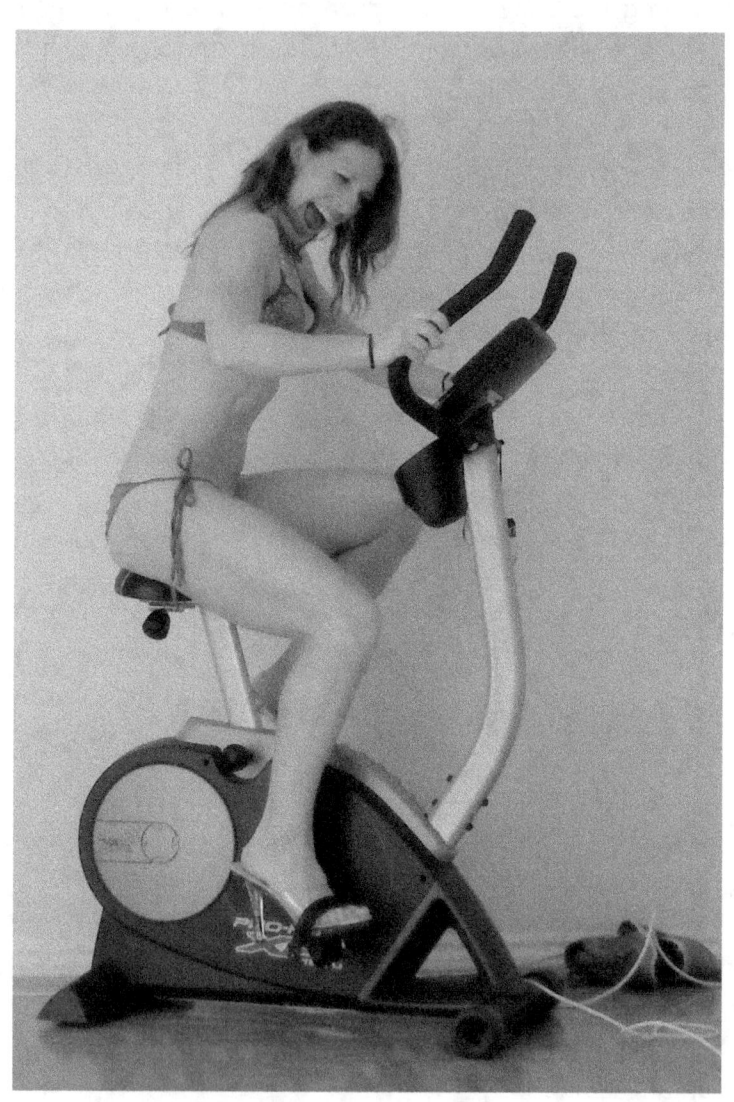

www.ingramcontent.com/pod-product-compliance
Lightning Source LLC
Chambersburg PA
CBHW062026280526

45787CB00005B/2230